ॐ

ॐ त्र्यम्बकं यजामहे सुगन्धिं पुष्टिवर्धनम्।
उर्वारुकमिव बन्धनान् मृत्योर्मुक्षीय मामृतात्॥

Drink Air Therapy To Kill Diabetes

A Path To Self-Cure And Immortality

Chandra Shekhar Kumar

Ancient Kriya Yoga Mission

Ancient Kriya Yoga Mission

ISBN-13: 978-1483912110
ISBN-10: 1483912116

Preface

Drink Air Therapy is an ancient practice for Self-Realization.

This book is written for preparing common mass to embrace a very simple but powerful self-help mechanism of drinking air(not breathing air) to eradicate Diabetes(both Type 1 and 2) from root and foster longevity with healthy body and mind.

Ancient Kriya Yoga Mission is engaged in disseminating simple techniques of ancient science of living.

These simple techniques are meant to be practiced by anyone without any external assistance and guidance.

For suggestions, feedback and comments, please send email to :
ancientkriyayoga@gmail.com

Ancient Kriya Yoga Mission

List of Chapters

List of Chapters

Chapter 1

Diabetes Mellitus

1.1   What is Diabetes Mellitus ?

Diabetes Mellitus is a metabolic disorder, leading to defective utilization of sugar by the body, which has plagued the mass since ages, increasing day by day as with the technological advancement of modern era.

Glucose is the major fuel for several bodily operations, organs and cells whose formation is done by the process of digestion due to breaking down of the dietary sugars and starch. The symptoms of diabetes are due to excessive sugar in the blood.

Glucose is controlled by the hormone insulin secreted by the organ *pancreas*. Whenthis gland is stressed enough or exhausted, the hormone insulin becomes deficient in quantity or sensitivity and the blood sugar level becomes high and uncontrollable as a result.

Diabetes is a very common disease today, especially in our affluent societies. Its incidence has paralleled the rising affluence of our lifestyle.

1.2 Main Symptoms of Diabetes

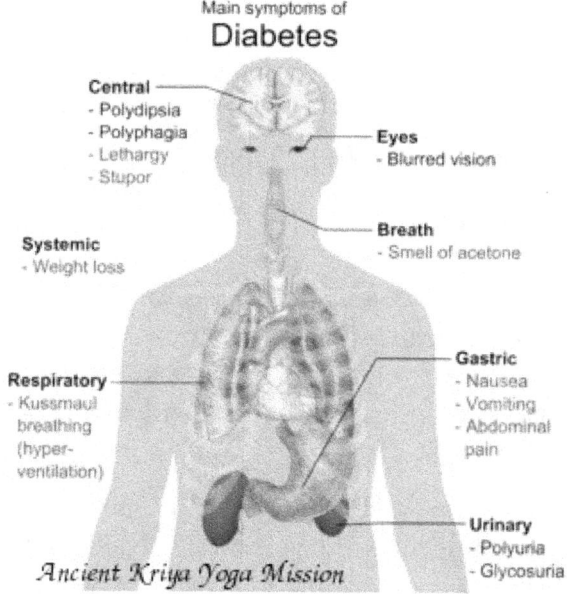

Main symptoms of
Diabetes

Central
- Polydipsia
- Polyphagia
- Lethargy
- Stupor

Eyes
- Blurred vision

Breath
- Smell of acetone

Systemic
- Weight loss

Respiratory
- Kussmaul breathing (hyperventilation)

Gastric
- Nausea
- Vomiting
- Abdominal pain

Urinary
- Polyuria
- Glycosuria

Ancient Kriya Yoga Mission

where *Polydipsia* is excessive thrust, *Polyphagia* is excessive hunger or increased appetite, *Polyuria* is excessive or abnormally large production or passage of urine and *Glycosuria* is the excretion of glucose into the urine.

Kussmaul breathing is a deep and labored breathing pattern often associated with severe metabolic acidosis, particularly diabetic ketoacidosis but also renal failure. It is a form of *hyperventilation,* which is any breathing pattern that reduces carbon dioxide in the blood due to increased rate or depth of respiration.

1.3 Main Cause of Diabetes

Diabetes mellitus is a chronic imbalance in the mechanism regulating blood sugar level.

When it occurs, the glucose absorbed into the blood from the digestive system is prevented from being effectively used in the muscles and tissues, or from being stored in the liver in the form of *glycogen* or as fat.

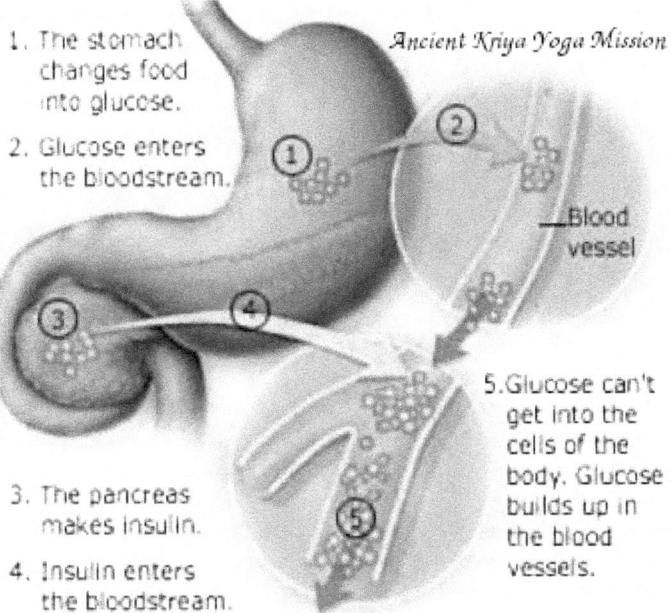

1. The stomach changes food into glucose.

2. Glucose enters the bloodstream.

Ancient Kriya Yoga Mission

Blood vessel

3. The pancreas makes insulin.

4. Insulin enters the bloodstream.

5. Glucose can't get into the cells of the body. Glucose builds up in the blood vessels.

As understood by now, it is caused either by a relative or absolute lack of the hormone insulin.

So its cause is attributed mainly to

1. lack of exercise and

2. *sedentary lifestyle.*

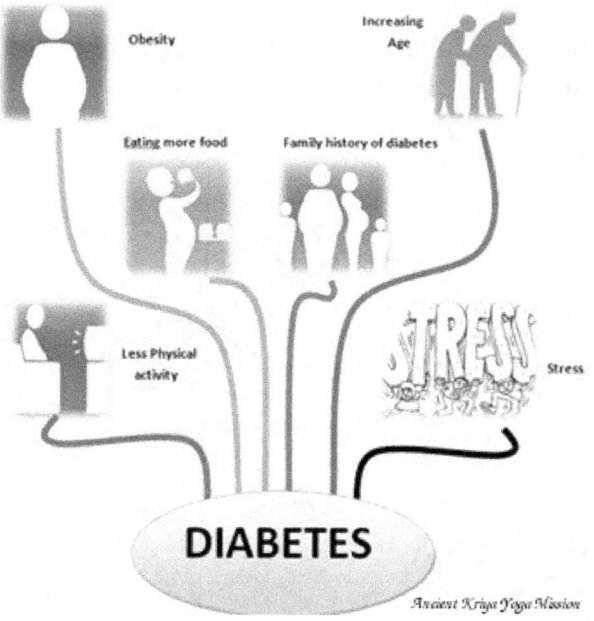

Ancient Kriya Yoga Mission

Type 1 Diabetes: Insufficient Insulin

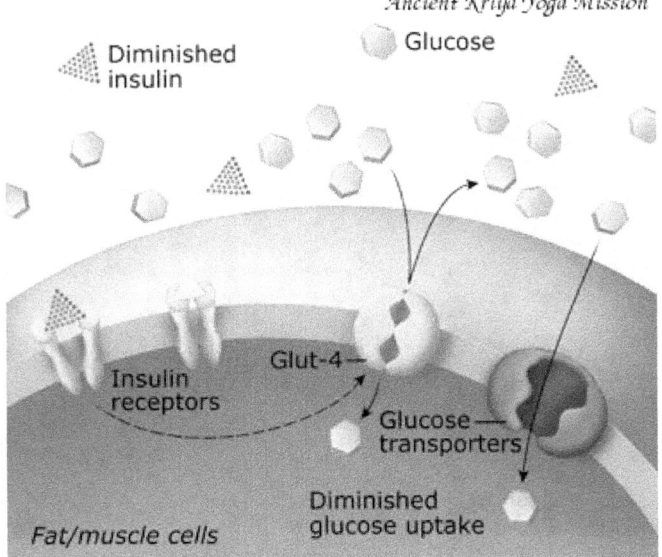

Type 2 Diabetes: Insulin Resistance

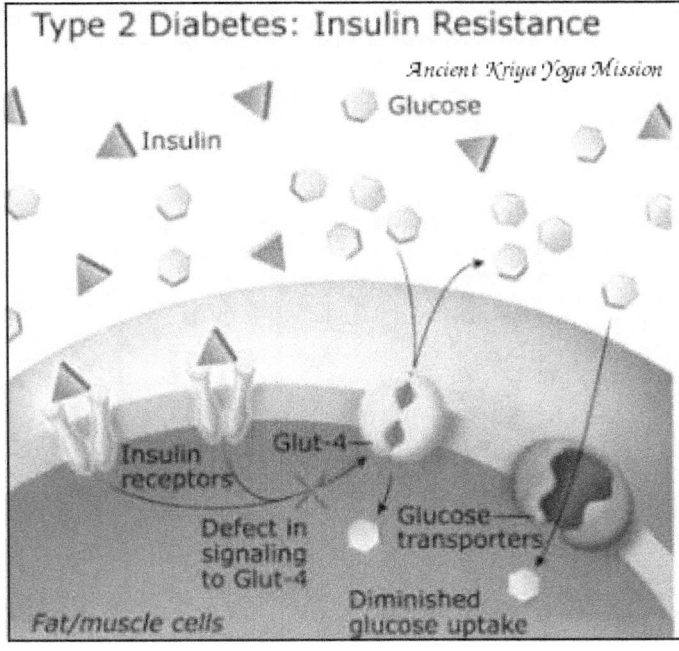

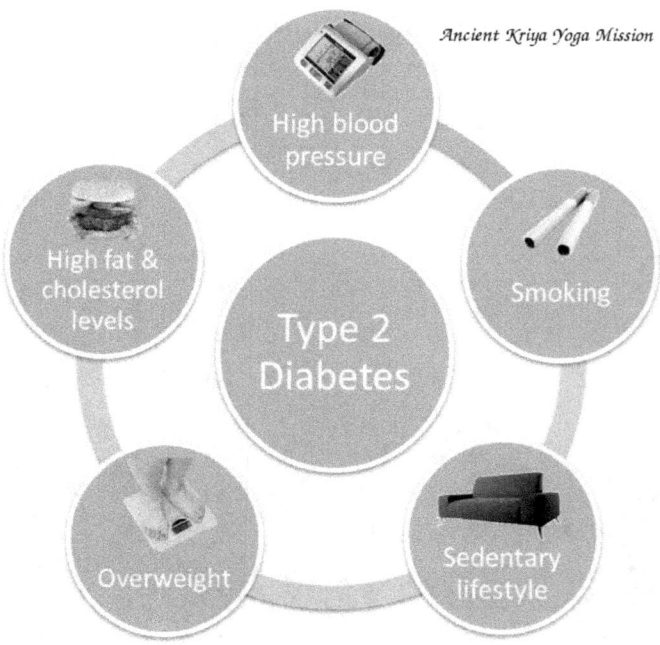

Ancient Kriya Yoga Mission

1.4   Glucose Metabolism

When we eat a meal containing protein, carbohydrate and fat, the following things happen in the normal situation:

1. Glucose enters the bloodstream from the intestines.

2. Insulin is then released from the pancreas in order to help the glucose from carbohydrates and amino acids from proteins to be assimilated by the body.

3. Insulin pushes the glucose into skeletal muscle, fat cells and liver.

4. Fat from the meal, in the form of triglyceride, is also pushed into fat cells by insulin.

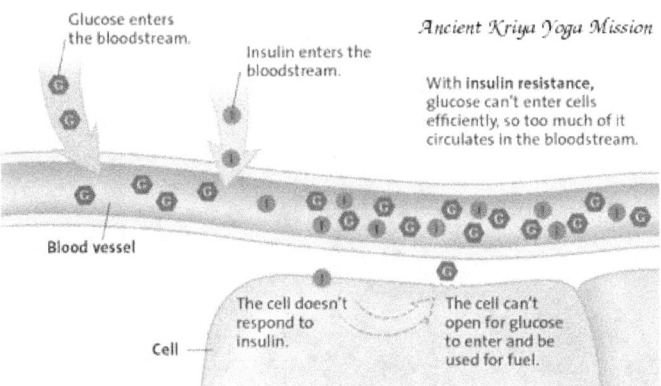

Because we do not eat continuously, periods of relative abundance alternate with food-free periods. During fasting the insulin levels reach their nadir and fat is released as a source of fuel. It is from this fat that ketones can build up to toxic levels in some people with diabetes.

The blood sugar regulates its own level. When the blood sugar level is high, the *Islets of Langerhans* secret insulin to lower the sugar level.

The opposite effect occurs when *Glucagon* is secreted. That's the right balance is achieved.

Islets of Langerhans is a group of endrocine gland cells in the pancreas with the specific function of secreting hormones.

Glucagon is another Islet cell hormone.

1.5 Insulin Production Cycle

Insulin is a hormone produced by the pancreas that is necessary for cells to be able to use blood glucose.

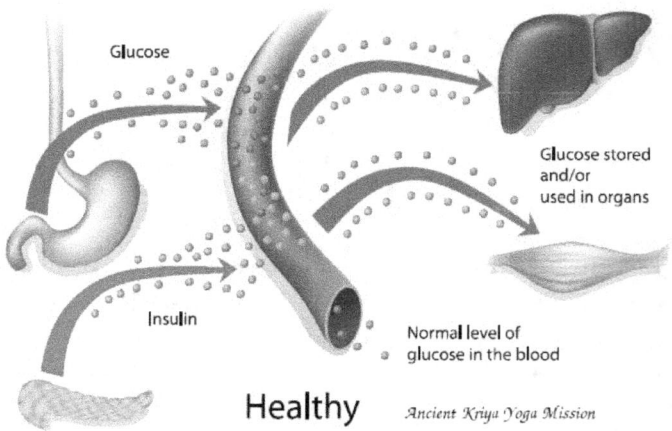

Glucose

Glucose stored and/or used in organs

Insulin

Normal level of glucose in the blood

Healthy *Ancient Kriya Yoga Mission*

In response to high levels of glucose in the blood, the insulin-producing cells in the pancreas secrete the hormone insulin.

Type 1 diabetes occurs when these cells are destroyed by the body's own immune system.

Diabetes mellitus is caused either by a relative or absolute lack of the hormone insulin.

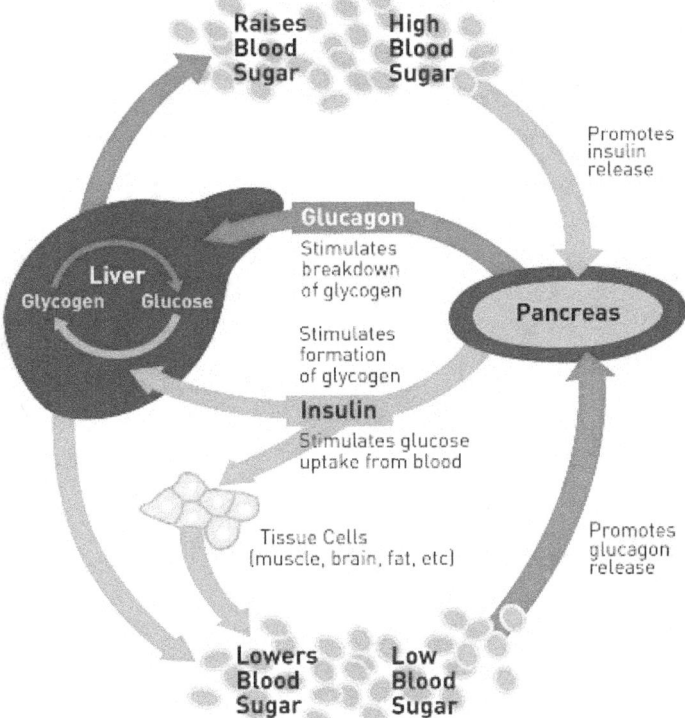

Ancient Kriya Yoga Mission

Diabetes mellitus is a chronic imbalance in the mechanism regulating blood sugar level.

When it occurs, the glucose absorbed into the blood from the digestive system is prevented

- from being effectively used in the muscles and tissues, or

- from being stored in the liver in the form of glycogen or as fat.

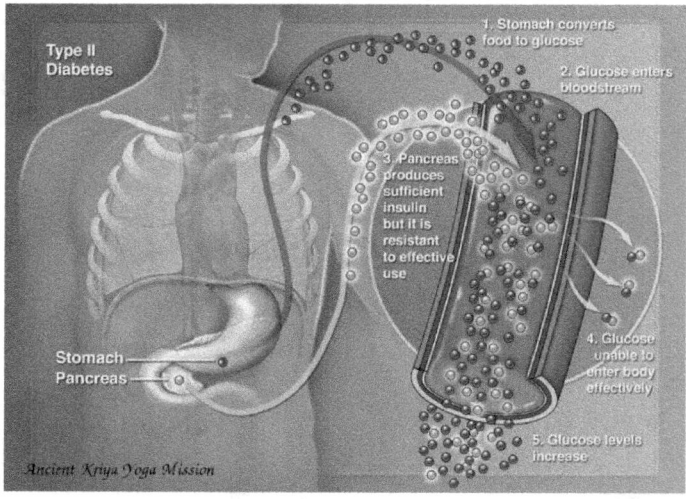

1.6   Challenge Ahead

The regulation of sugar by the body is a very complex process as glucose is the basic energy supplier of all body tissues. It plays an important role in all body functions and therefore requires sensitive and precise interaction of the pancreas, pituitary gland, muscles, liver, bloodstream, adrenal glands, thyroid gland, skin, kidneys and nervous system.

So glucose monitoring and control is a very complex process. It is now relatively easy to understand that diabetes is a very complex disease(or rather say disorder) and beyond the reach of medical therapy alone.

Chapter 2

Medical Therapy : A Vicious Circle

Diabetes Mellitus is a disease which has plagued man for centuries though its incidence at present, especially in the more developed areas of the world, is higher than it has ever been in the past.

The reason for this is that, through technological achievement, both stress and affluence have become increasingly widespread and people have developed the tendency to avoid strenuous physical exercise and to indulge in overeating.

Thus, the recent flourishing of diabetes, and diseases which stem from the same fundamental cause, can be considered to be a side effect of the twentieth century technological age, pollution on the personal level reflecting global pollution.

At the present time modern medical science holds that there is no positive system of cure for diabetes mellitus.

The most it can offer is control of the symptoms through dietary controls and daily use of insulin and other drugs. The disease itself, however is commonly not affected by this and may even increase in severity.

2.1 Type 1 Diabetes

In this condition for various reasons, the pancreas stops producing insulin. It can completely stop its production or it can dribble out insufficient quantities.

This prevents glucose from entering the body cells, with the result that they starve, even though there is a high level of food in the form of glucose in the blood stream.

This starvation affects the beta cells of the pancreas, compounding the problem and turning it into a vicious circle.

This form of diabetes most commonly occurs in young people.

2.2 Type 2 Diabetes

Due to malfunction or imbalance in the nervous, hormonal and digestive systems, there is thought to be an inappropriate secretion of insulin at the wrong time, and/or the body tissues have become less responsive to insulin.

In this form of diabetes, insulin release appears

to occur too late in the cycle, so the blood sugar level rises to a high level before insulin is secreted.

When insulin is finally liberated, there is not enough to cope with the high blood sugar level. The pancreas tries to secret more insulin, but it is too late, for by then the liver has started to release glucose in response to the call from the starving blood cells. Thus the level of sugar in the blood rises even higher.

In addition to this, the insulin that is released may be ineffective in letting the glucose into the cells because the cells themselves can not take it in or because insulin is poorly manufactured.

There are various degrees of this type of diabetes, from mild to severe. Some cases are even latent. Factors involved in this type of diabetes seem to be heredity, increasing age, obesity, infections and stress.

2.3 Oxygen Sandwich

Oxygen Sandwich is considered one of the major advancement of medical science to boostify the production of *stem* cells.

Islet Cell Transplantation is seen as the best hope for a cure for patients with *Type 1 Diabetes*, but there are still major challenges to be addressed, namely, the shortage of donor tissue supply since patients often need a reinfusion of islet cells after the initial treatment, and this means another donor pancreas is needed to provide the fragile cells for transplant.

To alleviate some of these problems, UM Researchers created a new cell culture device called the *Oxygen Sandwich* to provide the cells with a more natural oxygen environment than those used in traditional methods.

This device sandwiches the stem cells with oxygen from two sources :

1. one from the top with air diffusing through the culture medium and

2. the second from the bottom with air diffusing through a silicon membrane mixed with perfluorocarbon, a very powerful oxygen reservoir.

The use of high oxygen to promote differentiation of insulin-producing cells opens the way to many other progenitor cells, beyond embryonic stem cells and beyond diabetes.

Chapter 3

Drink Air Therapy for Beginners

3.1 Introduction

The ancient science of yoga has a more success-
ful method of management which is thousand of
years old.

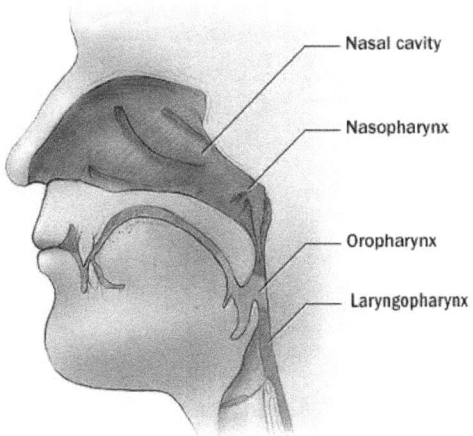

It is based upon the *internal readjustment* of the physical organism through *stimulation of the body's own regenerative processes.*

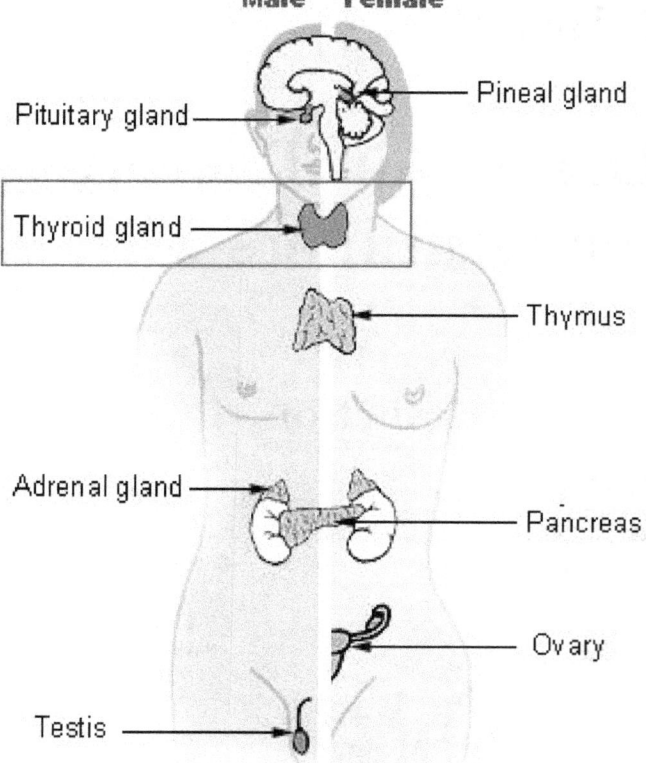

Major Endocrine Glands

Ancient Kriya Yoga Mission

After many years of successfully dealing with sufferers of diabetes through implementing the integral yogic system, we wish to make the knowledge of these efficacious techniques available to all interested sufferers and therapists of diabetes of the world.

3.2   Simplified One month program

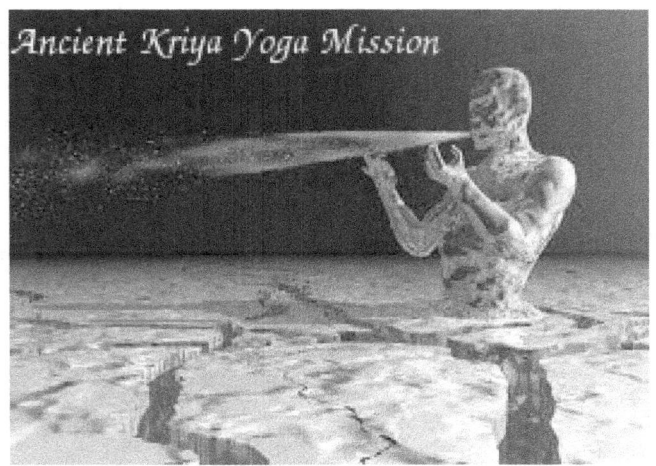

1. Sit is a comfortable pose.

2. Hold the head and back straight.

3. Close the eyes. Relax the whole body.

4. Fix your concentration on the place between your eyebrows.

5. Inhale slowly through both nostrils, preferably for 6 seconds for one slow inhalation.

6. Exhale slowly through both nostrils, preferably for 6 seconds for one slow exhalation.

7. One inhalation and one exhalation cycle cost together 12 seconds. So in a minute 6 inhalation plus exhalation is executed.

8. Repeat the above for 10-15 minutes.

9. Practice the above 2 times a day for 1 week.

10. Once comfortable in the above technique, start breathing air through your mouth as well as if you are drinking air taking 6 seconds for inhalation and 6 seconds for exhalation.

11. Repeat the above for 10-15 minutes.

12. Practice the above 2 times a day for 1 week.

13. Once the above technique is mastered, try to inhale and exhale by just using mouth.

14. Insist on drinking air as if taking gulps of air in chunks.

15. Repeat the above for 10-15 minutes.

16. Practice the above 2 times a day for 1 week.

17. Rate of drinking air should be reduced day by day, say, 4 seconds.

18. Repeat the above for 10-15 minutes.

19. Practice the above 2 times a day for 1 week.

Once the above schedule is finished, then try to drink air with similar or slower rate anytime anywhere while being comfortable.

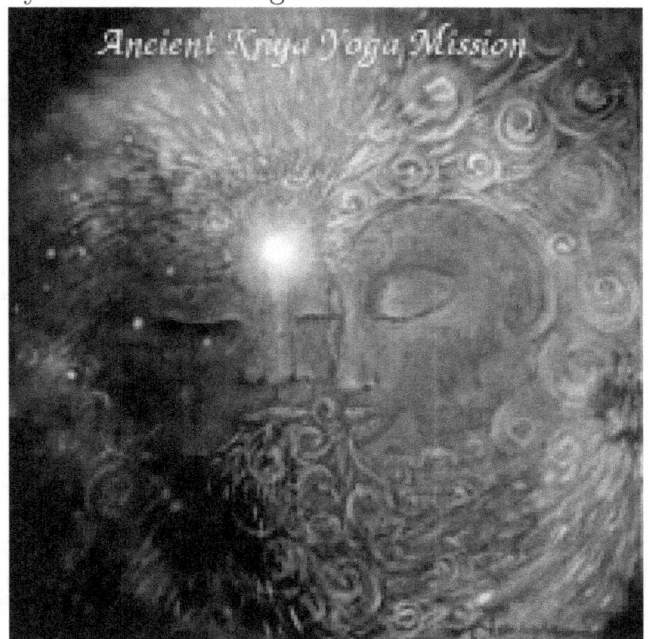

In general we can say that *Drinking Air Therapy* is helpful for all ailments that originate from nervousness or chronic stress.

Chapter 4

Advanced Drink Air Therapy

This is a unique form of *Drinking Air Therapy* in which one makes a hissing or whispering sound in the region of the throat. It is far easier to do than to describe.

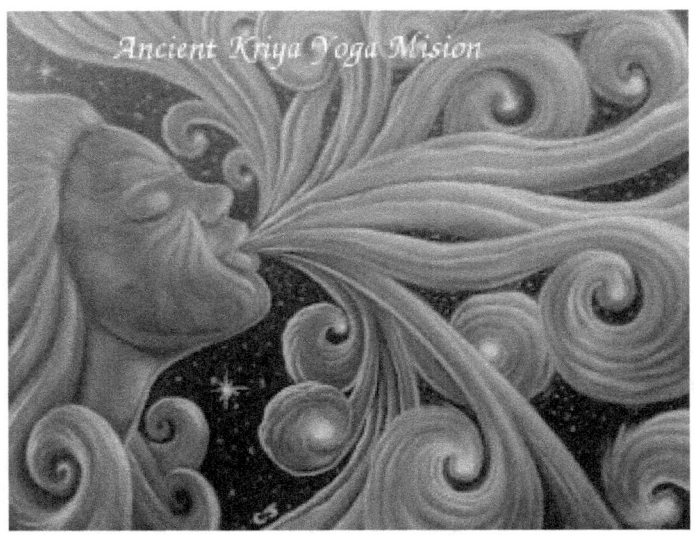

4.1 3 months program

1. Sit in any comfortable position.

2. Close the eyes.

3. Relax the body, holding the neck and head upright.

4. *Drink Air* slowly and deeply as described earlier.

5. Partially close the glottis in the throat. This is done by slightly contracting the throat.

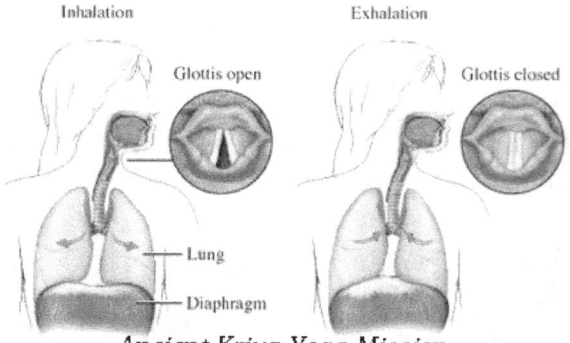

Ancient Kriya Yoga Mission

6. If this done properly you will simultaneously detect a slight contraction of the abdomen.

7. We are a little reticent about writing this fact down for it is easy for the practitioner to misunderstand and make a special point of contracting the abdominal muscles. *This should not be done.*

8. If you merely contract the glottis you will automatically feel a slight pulling sensation

in the region of the abdomen.

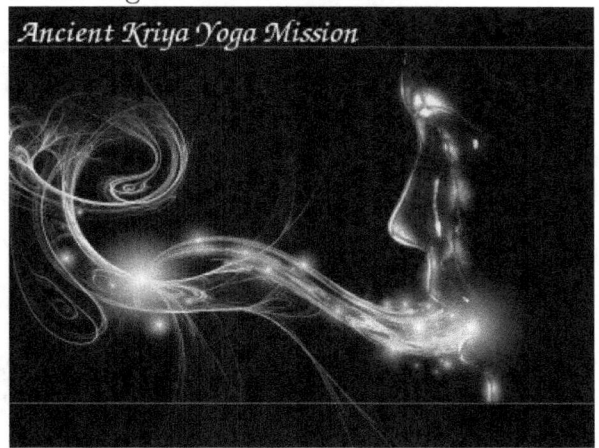

Ancient Kriya Yoga Mission

9. As you *drink air*, you should hear a continuous sound emitted from the throat.

10. It should not be very loud, audible just to yourself but inaudible to another person unless he sits very close to you.

11. This sound is caused by the friction of the air as it passes through the restriction that you have made in the glottis by contraction.

12. The sound will be similar to the gentle sound that a baby makes while sleeping.

13. It is possible that the practitioner is still not sure that he is doing this practice correctly. A similar contraction of the throat is obtained if you whisper aloud. Try to whisper aloud enough so that a person can hear you a few meters away. This should help indicate the method of contracting the glottis.

14. However, this is only intended an illustration and whispering should not be incorporated into *Advanced Drinking Air Therapy.*

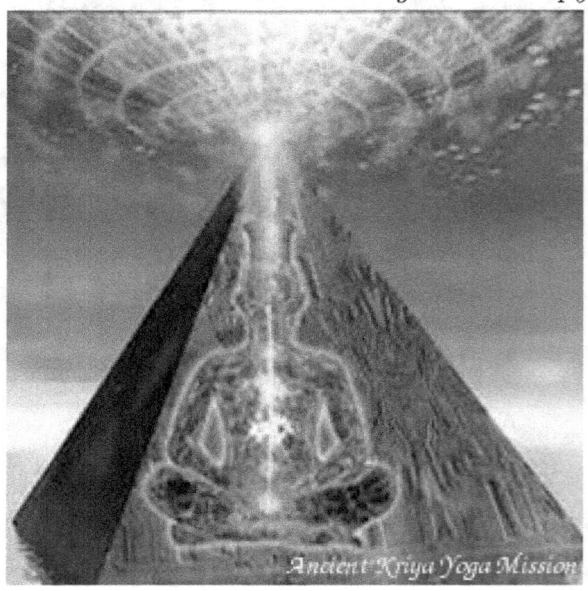

15. Many people contort their facial muscles when they are practicing *Advanced Drinking Air Therapy.* This is unnecessary. Try to relax the face as much as possible.

16. Do not over-contract the throat. The contraction should be light and applied continuously throughout the practice.

17. Keep your focus(while eyes closed) on the region between your eye brows. Keep *Drinking Air* slowly, smoothly and deeply, tending towards a rate of 4 in one minute.

18. Continue for 15-30 minutes in a go, twice or thrice a day, preferably empty stomach, for initial first month.

19. As you become comfortable with this practice, start practicing it anytime anywhere as much as you can for another 2 months, increasing the duration day by day.

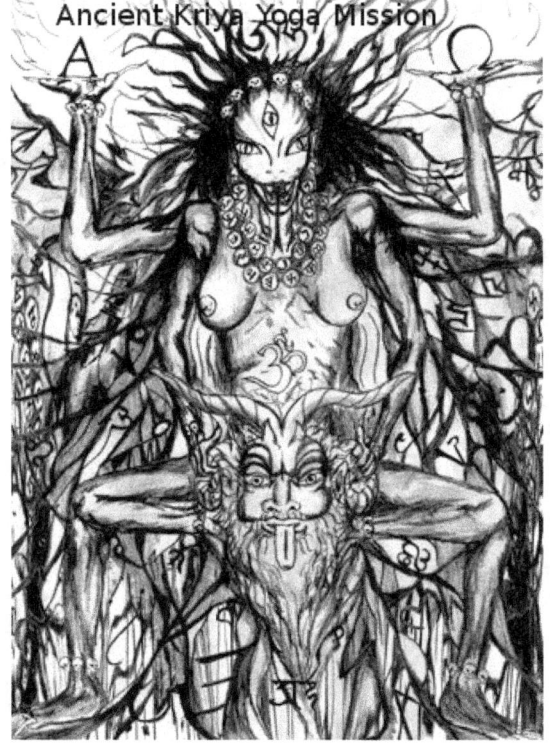

Ancient Kriya Yoga Mission

20. Part of one's awareness should be on the sound emerging from the throat and the corresponding inhalation and exhalation sandwiched with *Drinking Air.*

4.2 Benefits

Continued practice of this therapy results into significant decrease in metabolic parameters, namely

- fasting blood sugar

- post prandial blood sugar

- HbA1C

- lipid profile

and equanimity in the anthropometric measurements like weight, Body Mass Index, Waist-hip ratio.

There are significant decrease in the total cholesterol, triglycerides and low density lipoprotein levels.

It has already proven its mettle in the improvement of oxidative stress as well as in improving the glycaemic status of diabetics through neuroendocrinal mechanism.

It directly rejuvenating cells of pancreas as a result of which there may be increase in utilization and metabolism of glucose in the peripheral tissues, liver and adipose tissues through enzymatic process. It results into a decrease in the drug requirements as well.

The beneficial effect on the insulin kinetics may be by improving the sensitivity of the target tissues thus decreasing insulin resistance and consequently, increasing peripheral utilization of glucose.

It results into a significant increase in insulin sensitivity and decrease in insulin resistance by reporting a significant rise in the number of insulin receptors following yogic-intervention.

In general we can say that *Advanced Drinking Air Therapy* is helpful for all ailments that originate from nervousness or chronic stress.

Chapter 5

Conscious Breathing

5.1 Alternating Breath

Let us observe our breath and the manner in which the air flows in and out of the nostrils.

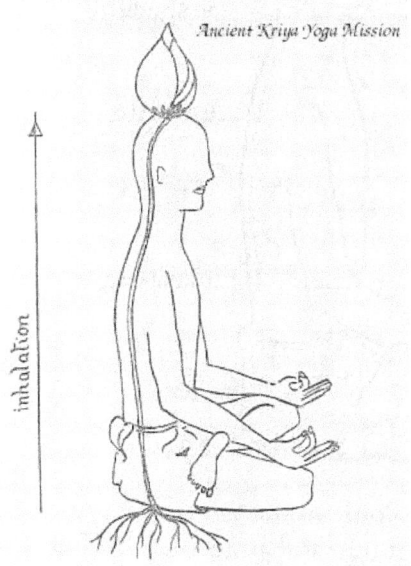

We notice that most of the time respiration takes place through one nostril only.

It appears that respiration occurs through both nostrils simultaneously, but this is not so.

When we observe the breath, we find that one nostril usually remains open for a certain duration of time and the breath comes and goes through that side only. Later this nostril closes and the alternate nostril opens. Every hour or every and twenty minutes the active nostril changes.

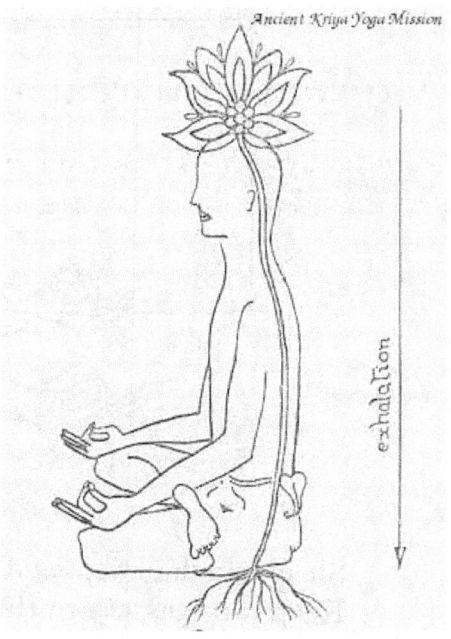

This rhythm regulates all the psychological and physiological processes. Physiologically, it has a particular effect on the nervous system, producing a certain type of stimulus. Furthermore, it has a specific influence on the brain which requires very systematic regulation.

5.2 Three Breaths

In fact, this is not just by chance that the breath flows sometimes though the right nostril and at other times through the left.

The rhythm of the body is based on the biorhythms, the energy rhythms of the body and it also relates to the two hemispheres of the brain.

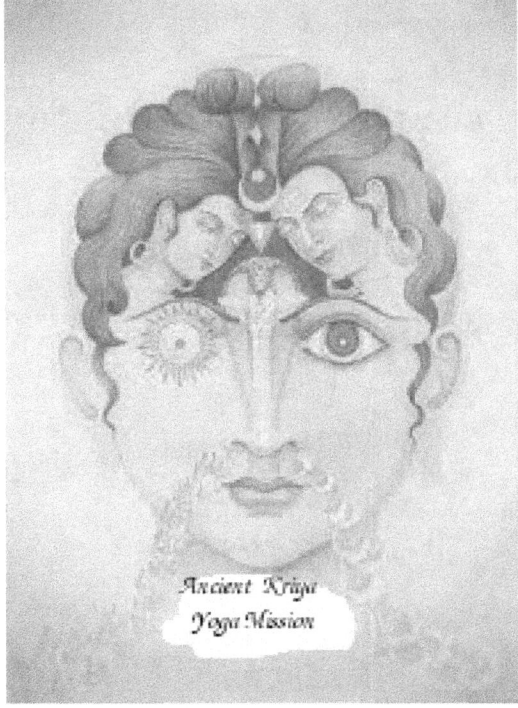

1. *Mental Breath* : Breathing from left nostril. Controls right hemisphere. Labeled as cool-

ing, relaxing and introverting.

2. *Physical Breath* : Breathing from right nostril. Controls left hemisphere. Activates the physical body and externalizes awareness. Labeled as heating, energizing and extroverting.

3. *Balanced Breath*: Breathing from both nostrils. It transcends the barrier of subject and object, i.e. body and mind. One enjoys life beyond empirical realm.

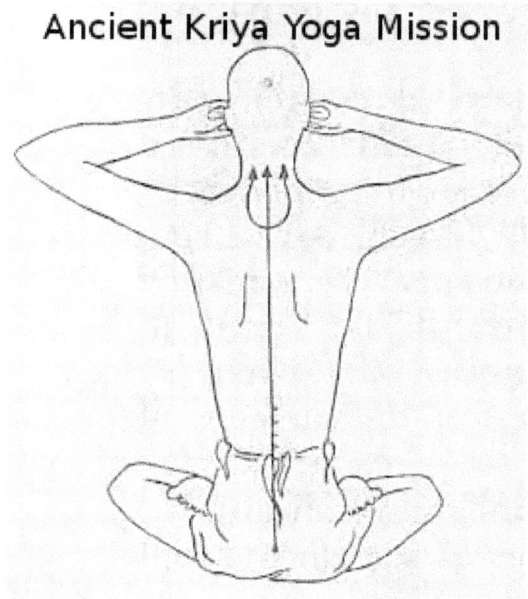

Ancient Kriya Yoga Mission

The specific functions of the cerebral region of the brain also correlate with the activities of *breathing*. The cerebrum is symmetrical, consisting of the right and left hemispheres.

The right hemisphere governs the left side of the body and the left hemisphere governs the right side of the body.

In the left hemisphere, information is processed sequentially, linearly and logically, thus making it suitable and responsible for rational, analytical and mathematical ability.

Conversely, the right hemisphere processes information in a diffuse and holistic manner. It controls orientation in space and is particularly sensitive to the vibrational realm of existence and those experiences which are intangible to the external sense receptors.

Thus the right hemisphere is responsible for psychic and extrasensory perception, and stimulates creative, artistic and musical abilities.

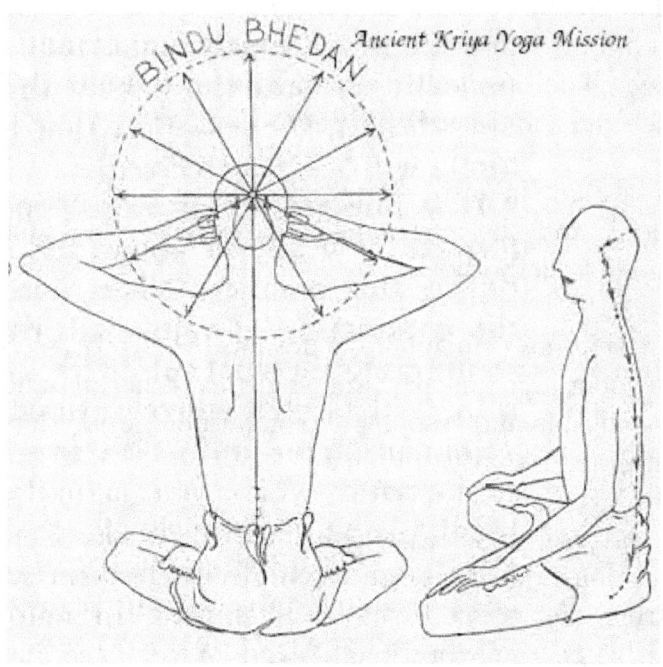

5.3 Guided Approach

While medical science claims that diabetes is incurable, many studies have proven that it responds very well to yogic management.

In clinical trials, newly diagnosed diabetics have reduced blood sugar to normal levels and insulin dependent diabetics have been able to either discontinue insulin usage completely or have been able to considerably reduce their insulin consumption.

The newly diagnosed diabetic has excellent

prospects of completely controlling and correcting his condition if he adopts yogic practices and lifestyle under guidance.

There is various yogic exercises and techniques to alleviate these ailments and lead the practitioner towards a healthier lifestyle.

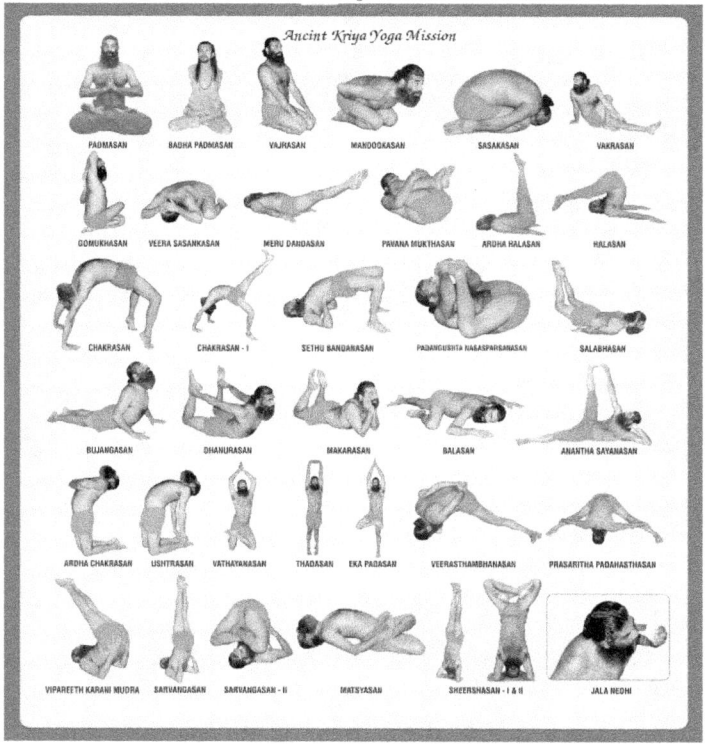

Because many of these techniques indeed demands attention of an *adept*, availability of which cannot be guaranteed always, that's why we advocate *Drinking Air Therapy* because it doesn't require any specific guidance by an adept. It can be practiced by an individual on its own with out any negative side effect.

Chapter 6

Cosmic Drink(Nectar)

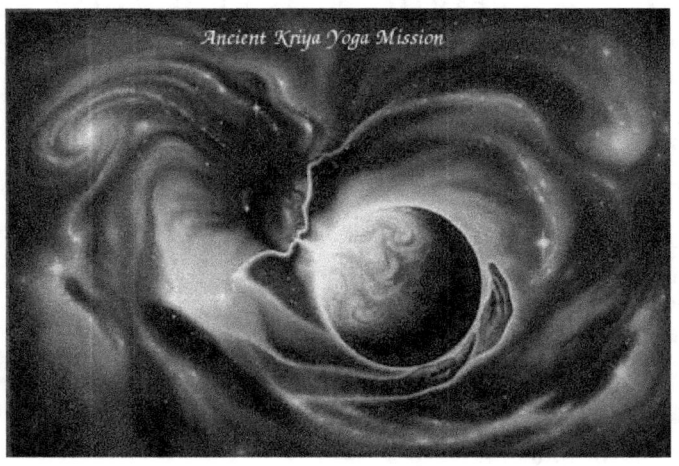

Practice the following schedule daily at least 2 times, preferably empty stomach.

6.1   Initial Preparation

1. Sit in any comfortable position with the head and spine straight.

2. Relax the whole body and close your eyes.

3. Focus your attention at the tip of your nose.

4. Practice *Drinking Air Therapy* as mentioned earlier for 10-15 minutes.

This has to be continued for 1 week before moving on the next step.

6.2   Straightening Tongue

1. Roll out your tongue.

2. Stretch the tip of the tongue forward and straight comfortably and maintain this position for 2-3 minutes.

3. Repeat this at least 2-3 times.

4. Keep *Drinking Air.*

This has to be continued for 1 week before moving on the next step.

6.3   Stretching Tongue

1. Stretch the tip of the tongue upward towards the tip of your nose.

2. Maintain this position for 2-3 minutes.

3. Repeat this at least 2-3 times.

4. Keep *Drinking Air*.

This has to be continued for 2 weeks before moving on the next step.

6.4 Fixing Tongue on Nose

1. Try touching the tip of your nose while being as much comfortable as possible.

2. Station your tongue on the tip of your nose.

3. Maintain this position for 1-2 minutes.

4. Repeat this at least 5-6 times.

5. Keep *Drinking Air*.

This has to be continued for 4-6 weeks before moving on the next step.

6.5 Bending Tongue

Ancient Kriya Yoga Mission

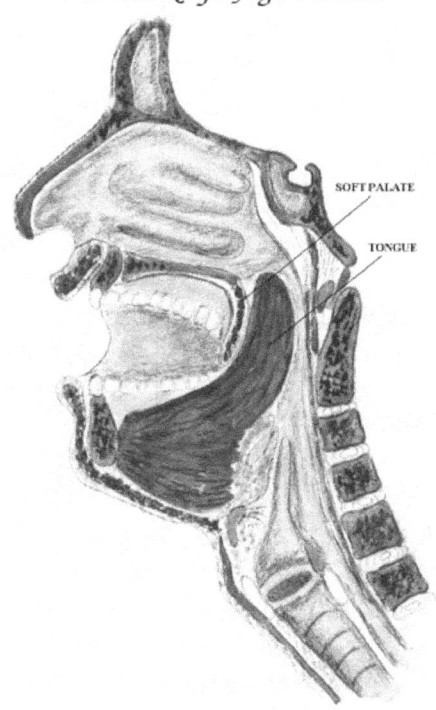

SOFT PALATE

TONGUE

1. Fold your tongue upward and backward so that the lower surface lies in contact with the upper palate.

2. Stretch the tip of the tongue backward as far as possible while being comfortable.

3. Maintain this position for 1-2 minutes.

4. Repeat this at least 5-6 times.

5. Keep *Drinking Air.*

This has to be continued for 8-12 weeks before moving on the next step.

6.6 Drinking Air Rate

At first there may be some discomfort and *Drinking Air* may irritate the throat, but with practice it will become more comfortable.

When the tongue becomes tired, release and relax it, then repeat the practice as mentioned.

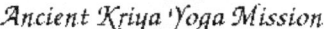

Ancient Kriya Yoga Mission

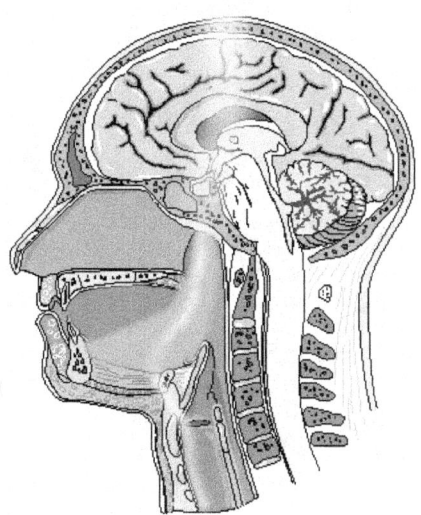

At first the rate of *Drinking Air* will be normal, i.e., 15-16 times a minute, but with gradual practice over a period of 3-4 months, it will come down to 5-6 times a minute.

This may be reduced further under the guidance of a competent instructor.

6.7   Stages

In the beginning stages and applicable for most practitioners, the tip of the tongue touches the soft palate as far back as possible without straining or placed in contact with the uvula at the back of the mouth.

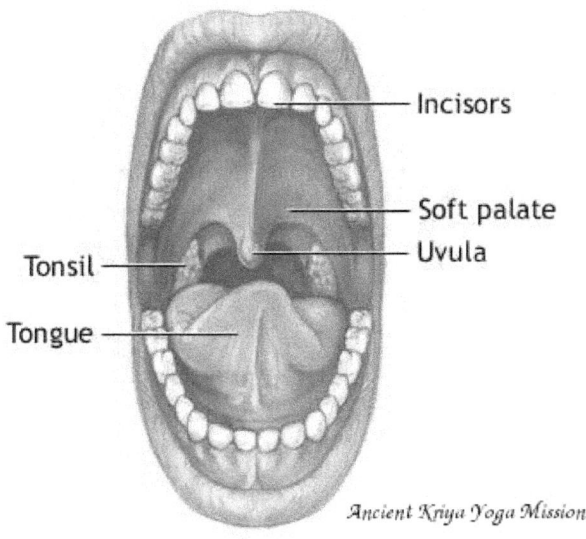

Ancient Kriya Yoga Mission

This practice has mainly 4 stages as can be depicted as:

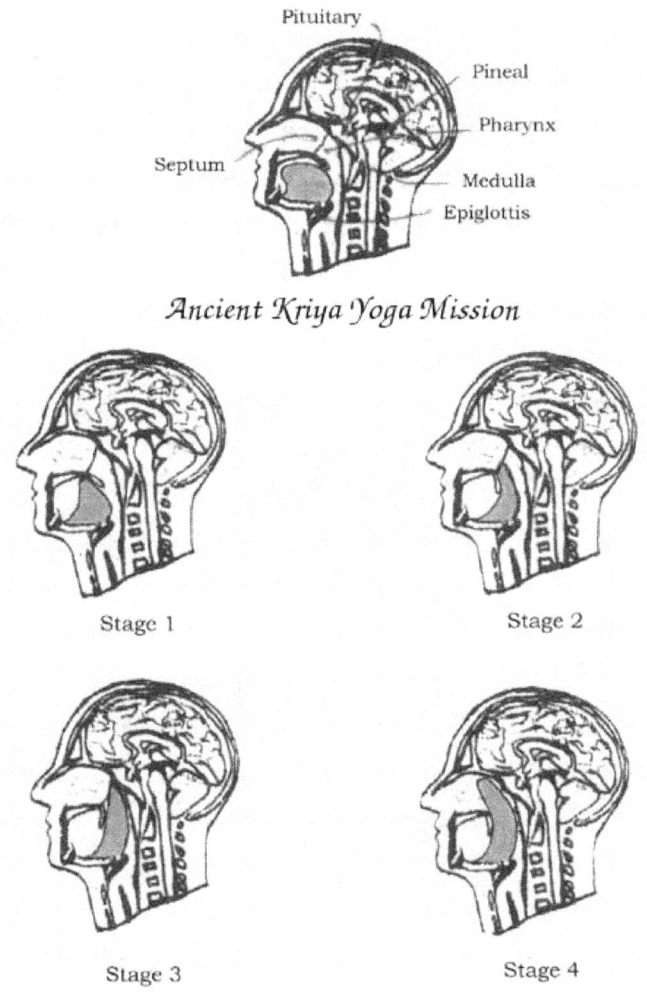

Ancient Kriya Yoga Mission

Stage 1   Stage 2

Stage 3   Stage 4

6.8   Understanding It

In the neck there are two remarkable organs called the *carotid sinuses* situated on each side of the main artery supplying the brain with blood, in front of the neck and just below the level of the jaws.

These small organs help to control and regulate blood flow and pressure. If there is any fall in blood pressure, it is detected by these two sinuses and the relevant message is sent directly to the brain center.

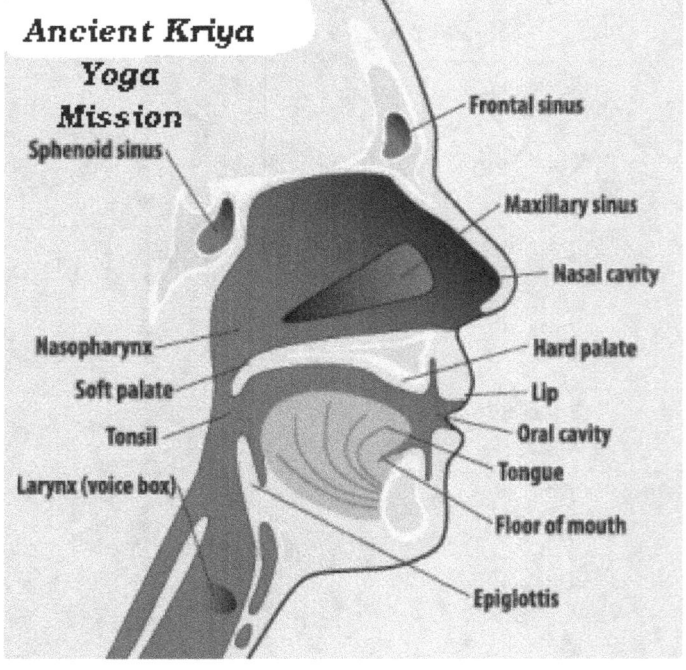

The brain responds immediately by

- increasing the heartbeat and

- contracting the arterioles(tiny blood vessels)

This results into raising the pressure to its normal level.

Any rise in blood pressure is also detected by the

carotid sinuses, which inform the brain and the opposite steps are performed to rectify and control the situation at hand.

Tension and stress are associated with high blood pressure. *Drinking Air Therapy* by applying a slight pressure on these sinuses in the neck causes them to react as though they have detected high blood pressure, with the result that the heartbeat and the blood pressure are reduced below normal. One becomes physically and mentally relaxed. It reduces overall relaxation, which is essential for success in killing diabetes.

Cosmic Drinking accentuates this pressure in the throat region and consequently on the two carotid sinuses.

It is a very simple practice but it has many subtle influences on the body and brain, both physical and mental as well as bioplasmic. The slow and deep drinking results in immediate calmness of the mind and body, as well as bringing the bioplasmic body into harmony.

6.9 Advantage

As we have already said that this practice bestows several benefits and it is usually practiced in this way. However, those people who merely want to relax themselves can apply *Drink Air Therapy* for just 10-15 minutes daily.

People who suffer from insomnia will find it especially useful. Those who suffer from high blood pressure will find that *Drinking Air* helps to reduce blood pressure, even if only for a short period of time at first. However, during this period the body and mind will gain much needed rest.

In general we can say that *Cosmic Drinking* is helpful for all ailments that originate from nervousness or chronic stress.

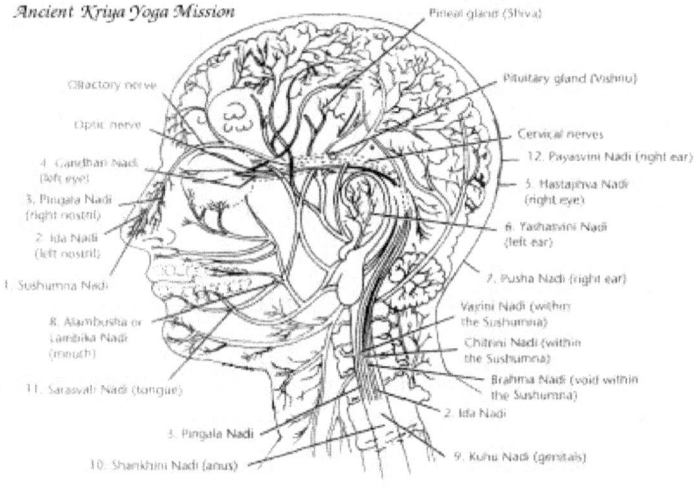

Ancient Kriya Yoga Mission

Pineal gland (Shiva)

Olfactory nerve

Optic nerve

4. Gandhari Nadi (left eye)

3. Pingala Nadi (right nostril)

2. Ida Nadi (left nostril)

1. Sushumna Nadi

8. Alambusha or Lambika Nadi (mouth)

11. Saraswati Nadi (tongue)

3. Pingala Nadi

10. Shankhini Nadi (anus)

Pituitary gland (Vishnu)

Cervical nerves

12. Payasvini Nadi (right ear)

5. Hastajihva Nadi (right eye)

6. Yashasvini Nadi (left ear)

7. Pusha Nadi (right ear)

Varini Nadi (within the Sushumna)

Chitrini Nadi (within the Sushumna)

Brahma Nadi (void within the Sushumna)

2. Ida Nadi

9. Kuhu Nadi (genitals)

Major Nadis in the head

6.10 Nature's Gift

Nature has blesses both man and frog with the ability to accomplish this.

Man is naturally in this position for nine months during the time when he stays in the womb. Here the child does not need to drink air as he is already cosmically drinking air.

Nature's unique gift to a newly born is that soon after birth, the tongue rolls down into normal position, as seen throughout life. The *Cosmic Drinking* comes to an end. the minute it ends, the process of normal breathing starts and the newly born starts crying, giving an indication of normalcy.

At times the tongue engaged in *Cosmic Drinking* does not unfold and the baby does not cry. Nurse or midwives are cautious to unfold the tongue by bringing the child's tongue back to normal position with their finger or by holding the child gently in an upside down position, patting lightly on his back, near the neck or around his forehead so that the tongue rolls back into position, and the child starts crying. If the child does not cry soon after birth, the above precautions nust be taken to avoid any serious harm.

The unique feature of *Cosmic Drinking* is that the baby does not need to breathe but receives nutrition. It is important for the baby to remain in *Cosmic Drinking Mode* for as long as he is in the womb. The tongue should displace itself from the prescribed position only after birth. As long as the tongue rolls down to normal position, need to breathe arises which is not possible in the womb. The result would be fatal for the child.

Nature has endowed the frog also with *Cosmic Air Drinking.* Man is in this state for a period of nine months only in the womb but a frog is blessed with this state all his life, intermittently.

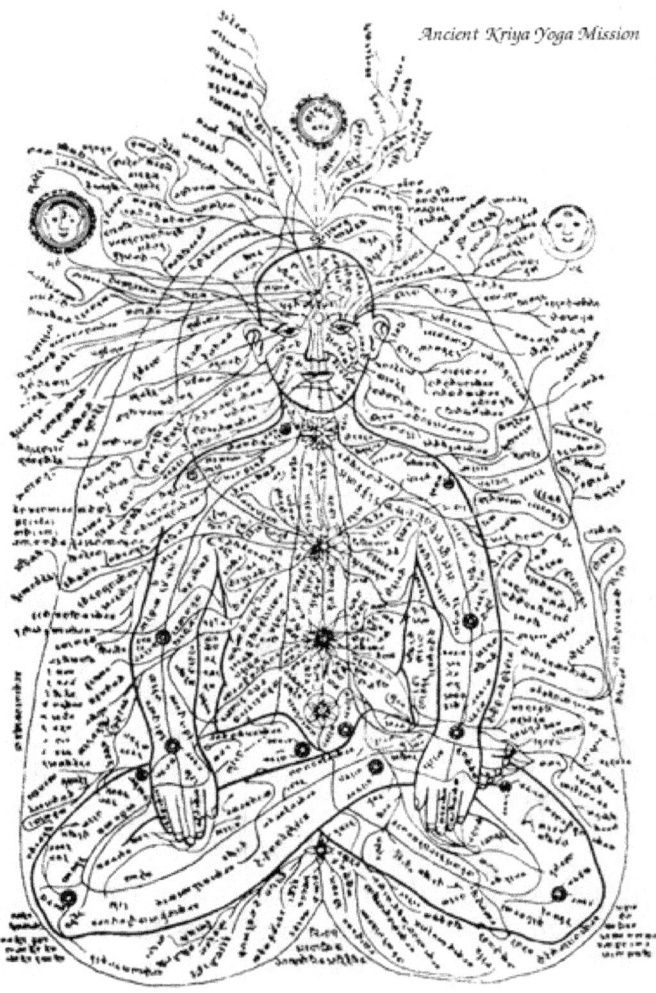

Ancient Kriya Yoga Mission

A frog can perform this therapy at any time. It has been observed that soon after the rainy season, frogs go underground when the weather turns inclement. While underground for a period of six to nine months it is in the state of *Cosmic Air*

Drinking foregoing the need to eat and breathe. As soon as rainy season starts, it emerges as its *Cosmic Air Drinking* comes to an end. This is repeated all its life.

Medical science calls this activity *hibernation.*

We at *Ancient Kriya Yoga Mission* are pretty confident that globalization of *Drinking Air Therapy* will enable common mass to lead a life free of disease, only then the true self-inquiry can began with ease.

Hari Om Tat Sat